Herbal Antivirals

How to Cure Illness with Holistic, All Natural, Herbal Medicines and Remedies

Table Of Contents

Introduction

First of all I would like to thank and congratulate you for downloading this book. This book is full of information about herbal medicines and how plants can help our health in natural ways.

Herbal remedies are the most common form of alternative medicine, and are widely used by people from all different cultures. Throughout history, herbs have also been seen as a legitimate form of medicine for treating all kinds of medical problems - from coughs and colds to digestive problems and skin conditions.

We have our ancestors to thank for herbal medicine - they are the ones who discovered the medical wonders that can be accomplished using only natural products. It is thanks to their findings that we have any of the drugs that we do today.

This ebook will explain all that there is to know about the history of herbal medicine, uses of herbal medicine, and recipes for some basic herbal remedies that you can make   at   home.

Chapter 1 – Herbal Remedies that Boost and Repair the Immune System

The immune system is our body's defence system against infections and diseases. The cells in the immune system have the ability to remember the diseases that they have encountered before and produce antibodies to defend the body from another attack. When the immune system is compromised we become vulnerable to diseases. To encourage a strong immune system we must have a healthy active lifestyle, plenty of rest and sun and little or reduced stress.

In order to have a healthy immune system when a healthy lifestyle is out of our reach, sometimes supplements can be taken. Traditional supplements are an option, but since these supplements are in forms of tablets and capsules some parts of it cannot be digested by the body. Some residues from the tablets can harm the kidneys because they are not being flushed out properly. In answer to that, herbs can be used to boost the immune system.

Here are some examples:

Astragalus is best known for stimulating the immune system. This herb from China also aids in digestion by lowering the acidity of the stomach. It is also commonly used for aiding the adrenal gland functions and fighting cold and flu. Astralagus' root can be in the form of tincture (a drinkable liquid substance), or in the form tablets or capsules. Astralagus is also known to heal wounds when applied topically to affected areas.

Bell peppers serve multiple purposes when it comes to herbal medications, They contain beta-carotene (which is converted to vitamin A), carotenoid lycopene (which lowers the risk of cancer), and Zeaxanthin (which prevents cataracts and macular degeneration).

Bell Peppers can be included in your everyday menu, in this way, you will be able to absorb Vitamin A from it.

Cat's Claw from Peru is commonly used for stomach problems, but is also becoming known for its oxindole alkaloids that stimulate the immune system and aid in fighting off infections and diseases. The bark and root of Cat's claw have attributes that help the immune system, increase the body's white blood cell count, and help internal organs to relax.

Echinacea is an herb used to prevent and treat respiratory tract infections and the common cold. Echinacea can be taken as tea, but people say it does not taste good so they often take it as a capsule or tincture. Echinacea is best taken as a tea or as a tincture, as they are more effective than capsules for ingesting the herb's active ingredients.

Ganoderma (also known as reishi) is a bitter mushroom that is popular in Chinese medicine for promoting longevity and health, combating cancer, and strengthening the immune system. It is often taken in the form of Ganoderna coffee, and has been shown to help immune system functioning, aid in weight loss and even combat cancer and diabetes.

Garlic is popular for its medicinal value and antiseptic, anti-microbial and cardiovascular properties. Despite its benefits, garlic must be avoided by mothers who are breastfeeding, as it has been known to make breastmilk taste bitter.

Ginger is known for its anti-inflammatory properties, its ability to reduce cardiovascular problems, and decrease cholesterol. There are many herbs and supplements that include ginger. Ginger is one medicinal herb that is much better to take as a supplement than to rely on its benefits by using it as an ingredient in everyday cooking.

Gingko Biloba's leaves contain antioxidants called gingkolides and bilobalides that defend the body from free radicals. Teas and tablets are available that have concentrated amount of gingko biloba, and it can be taken every day without any known side effects.

Ginseng. Korean ginseng has ginsenosides which give it anti-inflammatory and anti-cancer properties. Ginseng also boosts the immune system, psychological functions and other conditions related to diabetes.

Turmeric spice contains high amounts of curcumin, which is known for its antioxidant, anti-inflammatory, and antibacterial properties. Turmeric also aids digestion by stimulating bile flow.

These herbs are just a few of the herbs that can help you to boost your immune system. It is always safest to consult your doctor first before taking any of the above-mentioned herbs and supplements.

Chapter 2 – Herbal Antibiotics: Herbal Remedies that Kill Bacteria

An antibiotic is a drug that is used to treat infections caused by bacteria or other microorganisms. Many plants have antibiotic substances that are used to ward off infections, colds, flu, and also speed wound healing. Some herbs with antibiotic properties which also boost the immune system have already been mentioned, such as garlic and echinacea, but there are many others as well!

Here are some herbal antibiotics:

Acacia. Studies show that acacia extract has antibacterial activity that is highest in Staphylococci.

Aloe. Aloe has been found found to have high antibacterial activity against Staphylococcus aureus, Pseudomonos aeruginosa and herpes simplex. It is also widely used for treatment of burns.

Calendula is used to prevent infections, heal wounds and treat pink eye. It can be found in tincture, infusion, ointment or lotion form.

Cinnamon has antibacterial properties. It also aids in digestions and warms the body. It can be added to food, taken as a tea or used as an essential oil.

Cloves are used to kill bad intestinal bacteria. Cloves are also used as a topical analgesic and can be used as an essential oil or infused oil.

Licorice has antibiotic properties and also works against malaria.

Oregon grape root (when combined with Echinacea) can be a potential herbal antibiotic. That being said, it should not be taken by pregnant or breastfeeding moms.

Marshmallow root is often used topically to decrease pain, and heal and soften injuries. It also contains tannins, meaning that when it is made into a tea, it is effective in fighting bacteria in urinary tract infections.

Usnea is a common lichen used as both an antibacterial and antifungal, It also treats strep and staph infections, urinary tract infections, fungal infections and respiratory and sinus infections.

Yarrow flowers are crushed into powder, which can be used to stop bleeding completely. As well, when yarrow flowers are infused in water it speeds the healing of canker sores, and yarrow flower tea is used to treat urinary tract infections.

It is advisable to consult a medical expert first before taking these herbs, especially if you are considering taking these herbs as a substitute for a mainstream antibiotic.

Chapter 3 – Herbal Antivirals: Herbal Remedies that kill viruses

Viruses are small particles that cause all kind of health problems, such as the flu, the common cold and herpes. Treatment and prevention of viruses is an important issue. Incorporating natural antiviral herbs into your everyday diet is one of the best ways to treat and prevent common viruses. Most antiviral herbs have no side effects and are both cheap and safe to use. Some herbs with antiviral properties also have antibacterial properties and can be used to boost the immune system. These herbs include:astragalus, echinacea, garlic, ginger, cat's claw and licorice.

Here are some other herbal medicines that help to fight viruses:

African Potato improves the immune system and fights viruses.

Buchu is good in preventing viruses. This natural antiviral also has antiseptic properties and contains antioxidants that help to get rid of the body's toxins

Cranberries are full of antioxidants and are known for their antiviral properties. It is also used to treat urinary tract infections and used to fight plaque formation on teeth. Cranberries are best taken as a juice or in capsule form.

Elderberry leaves, roots, seeds and berries are used for viral infections like cold and flu. They also stimulate the circulation for sweating, which results in body cleansing.

Golden rod has been used for a hundred years as a traditional antiviral herb. It also increases the body's natural ability to fight infections.

Goldenseal is an immune booster and can be used as an anti-viral when combined with echinacea

Juniper is an anti-viral used to treat cold and flu viruses. It is commonly taken as a cold-season tea.

Lemon Balm served as a tea is an antiviral herb and is used to treat herpes.

Mullein is used as essential oil for ear infections and other ear problems when combined with garlic.

Olea Europea from olive leaves is a natural anti-viral that fights numerous germs. It has also been proven to boost the immune system

Onions, like garlic, are also an anti-viral herb. They can easily be added to most meals.

Oregano not only adds flavor to food but also defends the body against viruses and bacteria. It can be taken as an essential oil, as flavouring, or as a capsule.

Peppermint supports the body's immune system and is also an anti-viral herbs that treats tuberculosis. It can be used as essential oil or taken as tea.

Schizandra Sinesis is a Chinese herb that is used against viruses and protects against cell damage and other toxins

Shitake mushroom is an anti-viral herb which is also consumed in dishes and supplements.

Again, I cannot stress this enough, taking the time to consult with your doctor before taking any herbal treatments is always recommended. Self-diagnosing your problem is not safe in any way. While herbs may seem harmless, they have powerful medicative properties - and it is always better to be safe than sorry!

Chapter 4 –Herbal Remedy Recipes

Herbal remedies make use of antibacterial, antiviral herbs and herbs that boost the immune system. There are many different methods to prepare and use herbal remedies:

- A powder dissolved in hot water.

- Pastes taken with honey.

- Decoction (boiling the herbs for an hour or more)

- Teas

- Tinctures or herb extraction made with the help of diluted or pure spirits of alcohol.

- Poultices

- Capsulated forms.

Herbs can also be prepared and taken as an infusion, infused oil or tea.

Herbal Infusions

Herbal infusions are made from large quantities of herbs that are steeped for several hours and stored in a tightly sealed jar of water. This creates an incredibly concentrated solution that can be ingested orally or added to baths. Infusions are also commonly used for poultices and compresses.

Steps in making infusion:

1.   Put a handful of the dried herbs of your choice in a canning jar.

2.   Fill the jar with boiling water.

3.   Seal the lid of the jar tightly and let the mixture steep for four to ten hours

4.   Strain out the herbs. Use some of the infusion immediately, and store any excess in the fridge to slow spoilage.

Some suggested herbs for infusions include: nettle, oatstraw, red clover, comfrey leaf, alfalfa, dandelion, seaweed, clover blossoms, ginseng, and violet leaves. If you choose to drink your infusion as a tea you may want to add some honey or salt to help make the flavour more pleasant.

Infused Oil

Infused oil can be prepared for only few minutes. Here are the things you will need to prepare infused oil:

- Oven-proof dish

- Cheesecloth or strainer

- 1 cup coconut oil

- 1 cup herbs or combination of herbs

- Clean jars for storage

Process:

1. Preheat the oven to 200 degrees Fahrenheit, and then turn it off.

2. Mix the oil and herbs in the ovenproof dish

3. Leave the dish in the warm oven for three hours

4. Remove large pieces herbs by hand, and strain the rest of the oil into the clean jars.

5. Store your infused oils in a cool dark place.

Tea

Preparing tea is one of the simplest and most common ways of making an herbal remedy. All that is required is a cup, hot water, and the herb that you wish to use. Generally, it is recommended that you steep the 1 tbsp of the chosen herb in 1 cup of hot water for five to ten minutes. For a weaker dose, 1 tsp of herb in 1 cup of water is recommended.

It is important not to boil the herbs in the water, as this can destroy some of their medicinal properties. Some suggested herbal teas include: Bee Balm, Catnip, Chamomile, Coriander seeds, Lemon Balm, Fennel, Rose Petal, Mint, and Betony. If you are pregnant, you should check with your doctor before drinking most herbal teas (catnip tea, for example, is commonly not recommended for pregnant women).

While tea is the most common way to use herbal medicine, there are many other tips and tricks for natural healthcare. The rest of this chapter is dedicated to home remedy recipes that are very helpful in curing minor health problems. These recipes can be easily made at home from natural ingredients found in most kitchens or gardens.

Bug Repellant

Essential oils such as citronella, eucalyptus and lemon grass can be used to shoo away bugs. For adult use only.

Ingredients:

- 1 ounce witch hazel

- 3 drops of lemon grass essential oil

- 4 drops citronella essential oil

- 4 ounces distilled water

- 6 drops of lemon grass essential oil

Directions:

1. Mix essential oil in a metal or plastic spray bottle.

2. Shake well.

3. Add the rest of the ingredients and shake again.

Mixing this solution in a spray bottle allows you to apply the mixture evenly and easily, even to hard-to-reach areas of the body.

Eczema Relief

(For adults only)

Ingredients:

- 1 oz. Calendula oil
- 1 oz. Camelina oil
- 2 oz. Flax seed oil or Tamanu oil
- 2 oz. Emu oil
- 2 oz. Seabuckthorn oil

Directions:

Mix all oils together and pour into a small reusable bottle. Apply to the affected skin (avoiding the face) once or twice daily until eczema improves.

Cold and Flu Relief: Bath Soak

Ingredients

- 2 cups of Epsom salt
- 3 drops of eucalyptus essential oil
- 3 drops of rosemary essential oil

Directions:

1. Combine all ingredients
2. Pour mixture into stream of warm water as tub is being filled
3. Soak in tub for at least twenty minutes

Additional Benefits of Epsom Salt: The magnesium found in Epsom salt has been proven to lower blood pressure, reduce stress, improve mood, ease or prevent migraines, raise energy levels, provide pain relief and reduce muscle cramping.

Other herbal remedies for common ailments and illnesses:

Age spots:

Lemon juice or fresh lemon can be used to lighten age spots if applied regularly over a period of several weeks.

Arthritis:

Olive oil can be rubbed into the skin to relieve the pain of Arthritis or ingested through the diet - three tablespoons of olive oil is thought to be equivalent to a single ibuprofen in terms of anti-inflammatory effects.

Bee stings:

Make a paste using water and baking soda or toothpaste and apply to the affected area. The pain should be greatly reduced in ten minutes or less.

Burn Relief:

Turmeric root is known for its cholagogic and anti-inflammatory properties. Mix ¼ teaspoon of turmeric with 1 tablespoon of Aloe Vera and ¼ teaspoon of sandalwood and apply on affected area.

Carpal Tunnel:

Massaging peppermint oil and lavender oil into the skin surrounding the sore joints can help in relieving the pain of carpal tunnel.

Canker sores:

This natural remedy not only works, but also tastes great - helpful for sores on or around the mouth! Mix ¼ teaspoon turmeric with 1 teaspoon of honey, rub the paste onto the sore, and let it sit.

Cold Sores:

A mixture of tea tree oil and Aloe Vera helps to treat cold sores. Applying the mixture to the cold sore allows it to dry and heal quickly.

Headaches:

There are several herbs used to relieve headaches, including: violet, ginseng, orange peel, dandelion and Peppermint. These herbs are used in aromatherapy or made into tea and can act on their own or in combination to relieve headache pain.

Hiccups:

Hiccups will stop if you swallow a teaspoon of sugar with a few drops of water added.

Insect bite:

Create a paste that combines ½ teaspoon of turmeric powder and ½ teaspoon of sandalwood. Apply the paste to the bitten area to provide healing and soothing.

Poison Ivy or Poison Oak Relief:

Steep the roots and bark of the sassafras tree in one cup of boiling water for twenty minutes. Allow the resulting solution to cool. Make a strong cup of sassafrass tea and apply it to the affected area for several times a day. Do not rinse.

Psoriasis:

Tea tree oil is a very good remedy for all sorts of skin irritants. As well, Avocado oil works best on psoriasis if gently applied on the affected area.

Sunburn:

Milk is a very good sunburn remedy when applied to the affected area. You can also add 1/2 cup of baking soda to a cool bath for a calming effect on the skin.

Chapter 5 – Modern Vs. Traditional Medication

Traditional medicine and the use of herbalism is widely practiced all over the world, despite the fact that many who follow modern medicine believe that it doesn't consider enough scientific evidence. That being said, even modern medicine makes use of compounds derived from plants. The World Health Organization released a study which stated that a quarter of all modern day pharmaceuticals are wholly or partially derived from plants.

When deciding between traditional medication and modern medications, it is important to keep the following things in mind:

1. Traditional and folk remedy herbs are not without risks

People think that herbal medications are safer than modern pharmaceutical drugs or synthetic drugs because plants are 'all-natural'. While this may be true in some cases, herbs should be treated with respect and caution. Some herbs may still be associated with side effects when taken with other medications or may reduce or magnify the effects of modern drugs.

Here are some examples of possible herbal side-effects:

a. The herb Ephedra which is used as a weight-loss product and natural decongestant, may increase heart rate and blood pressure

b. Herbs used in combination with blood thinning pharmaceutical drugs may increase bleeding in patients, posing serious problems

c. St. John's Wort, often used to treat depression, may lessen the potency of other drugs taken with it

d. Medicinal herbs should not be mixed with alcohol or other recreational drugs as this can cause life-threatening side effects.

e. Herbs used to treat joint pain may result in mild hair loss, skin blisters, digestive disturbances, pus-producing infections or menstrual irregularity

f. Yellow oleander which is also called the friar's elbow is used for weight loss, and can cause vomiting and diarrhea and can damage the heart.

2. Herbal remedies lack quality assurance standards

Reports in recent years have shown that some herbal products are tainted with heavy metals and other dangerous contaminants. In some cases it has also been found that herbal products sometimes contain very little of the ingredients that they advertise, and sometimes do not contain any of the ingredient at all!

3. Taking herbs in pill form is better than eating the natural product

Active compounds like salicin (derived from the bark of the white willow tree) are sometimes isolated in pill form. Taking this herb in tablet form allows the active compounds to be administered in more precise dosage.

4. Isolating compounds may also have drawbacks

One possible drawback to isolating compounds from natural substances is that the active compound may lose some of its medicinal benefits. As well, the disease-causing organism can sometimes become resistant to isolated drugs. For example, quinine (from cinchona trees) can kill a huge percentage of malaria-causing parasites, but the parasites who do not die become resistant to quinine and become plentiful, and require additional medication to treat in order to combat the disease.

5. Combining Modern Western Medicine with Traditional Medicine can be beneficial

Many traditional herbal medications have been proven effective by doctors and pharmacologists. On a tour of a Chinese hospital, American pharmacologists were impressed by the evidence that some herbal medicines were effective with the nonsurgical treatments of gallstones, appendicitis and kidney stones. The mixture used to treat appendicitis is composed of magnolia, rhubarb, sargentoxoda genera and dandelion. While the Western world begins to adopt herbal medicines, Eastern medicine is now beginning to combine their traditional herbal treatments with the best of the Western modern medicine.

Chapter 6 – Prevalence of Herbal Medicine

One of the reasons that herbal medicine is so accepted in our culture today is because it has been used in all different cultures and nations for as long as civilization has existed. Almost every nation and culture have at one time used herbal medicine to treat various illnesses and diseases - even most pharmaceutical medications prescribed today have roots in herbal medicine! Understanding the rich history of herbal medicine is one of the most rewarding parts of entering into this

Herbal Medicine in Ancient Times

Recent archaeological discoveries have proven that people made use of natural herbs for healing purposes even thousands of years ago! In fact, some evidence of the use of medicinal plants dates back approximately 60,000 years ago to the Paleolithic era. Other significant cultures that have made use of herbal remedies include:

The Sumerians:

Written evidence shows a list of herbal remedies created by the Sumerians that dates back over 5,000 years ago.

Ancient Egypt:

The earliest recorded use of herbal medicine as a treatment for disease was written on the Ebers Papyrus in Ancient Egypt in the 16th century BCE. The papyrus contains hundreds of remedies using herbal medications for various afflictions. Some herbs commonly used in this time period were written or depicted in tomb illustrations and have been found in medical jars

Biblical times:

Hebrew physicians used remedies such as oil, balsam and wine to treat certain medical conditions. As well, poultices made from dried figs were used for treating boils.

Ancient Greece:

The work of the first century Greek physician Dioscorides appears to have begun the Western form of medical herbalism. Dioscorides wrote the book 'De Materia Medica' which became the leading pharmacological text for the next 1600 years. Other works which have survived from this era are those of

Krateus from the 1st century BCE and those of Diocles of Carystus from 3rd century BCE.

- •

Ancient China:

The use of herbal medicine in treating diseases has always been an integral part of Chinese history. Ancient folklore gave credit to the Yellow Emperor, Huang Di, for composing the Nei Jing, a collection of medical information. Medical practitioners in China still consult this canon of internal medicine when dealing with modern ailments. The canon explores many of the same subjects covered by a Western medical book - it discusses the symptoms, causes, diagnosis, treatments and prevention of diseases, as well as the anatomy and bodily functions affected by various herbs.

An ancient herb known as ginghao was reported to have been used in 341 C.E. The extract of ginghao, Asian wormwood, was believed to be a remedy for malaria. Its efficacy was rediscovered in the year 1971, when The Chinese Medical Journal reported that the herb was effective in tests on over 2000 patients.

Ancient India:

In ancient India, herbs were common as a form of medicine, especially as diet served as the principal treatment for disease in that time period.

Herbal Medicine in Recent History

In recent years, a number of global scientific studies demonstrate the widespread use of different herbs in treating modern diseases and conditions.

Asia and Africa:

80% of the population of Asian and African countries use herbal medicines according to World Health Organization.

Germany:

The use of traditional remedies continues to be popular in Germany. In fact, German government health programs even reimburse the cost of herbal prescriptions.

America:

American Indians often boil the roots of Black Cohosh - also known as black snake root, rattle root, or bugbane.

This solution is commonly used in connection with childbirth and menstrual problems. Recent studies by the Harvard Women's Health Watch of April 2000 suggest that the root extract may be effective in relieving menopausal syndrome.

China:

A visit with a Chinese doctor is quite different from a visit to a doctor in Western countries. A Chinese doctor usually sees patients from their place in an herb shop. There, the doctor of Chinese medicine (who is also the resident herbalist) will examine the patient, diagnose the medical problem and give an herbal prescription for treatment.

Recent news about a traditional herb used in treating rheumatoid arthritis comes from mainland China. Dr. Guo and his colleagues at Tianjin Hospital say that the root of the yellow vine has a therapeutic efficacy inferior only to steroids. Ninety eight percent of the patients who were given a daily dosage of the root, together with vitamin B tablets and other antacids have experienced relief of joint pains.

One of China's herbal preparations was also reported to cure or decidedly improve patients suffering from liver cirrhosis. This Chinese herbal medicine was developed from another medicine that is being used for treating chronic hepatitis.

United Kingdom:

Penelope Ody, a member of the National Institute of Medical herbalist in United Kingdom has written about more than 250 safe herbal treatments used to alleviate many common complaints ranging from ordinary headaches, colds, and coughs to illnesses that are much more severe.

Chapter 7 – Are Herbal Medicines Right for You?

Unfortunately, there are not any strict guidelines that will tell you whether or not herbal medicines will be the solution to your specific health problems. Certainly, if you are otherwise healthy choosing to try a few weaker recipes (such as the ones found in this book) can be an excellent way to start on your journey, and should not have any lasting negative effects. If you want to expand to other, more complicated herbal cures, be sure to do your research thoroughly before trialling anything!

If you have chronic health conditions, are pregnant, are currently on prescription medication, or are treating young children, it is wise to talk to your physician or healthcare provider before trying any form of herbal medication. While the medication itself may be helpful, there is always a chance that it will interfere with a previous prescription or health condition.

Herbal medicines can be a fantastic healthcare solution for those who want to boost their health while using natural remedies that can be grown in a household garden. Research is incredibly important as you begin this journey - there are many resources online, in-person, or in books that can help you to fully understand how best to administer herbal cures.

Conclusion

From centuries ago to modern times, from folklore to the modern medical practitioners, from North to South, and from East to West, traditional medication using herbs is becoming popular and accepted. Herbal medication is known to treat different illnesses and conditions from the most common problem like colds, flu or insect bites to more serious diseases, such as gall stones, cancer, and malaria.

Many people who use herbal antibiotics and antivirals believe that this strategy is more safe and effective than any other method. While there may be truth to this belief, herbal medication should be treated with both caution and respect. Some herbs may cause minor complications (like allergies) to severe complications - this means that it is very important to consult a skilled herbalist before trying to use herbs, especially if the patient has a complicated condition. Administering herbs with the correct dosage and frequency is also very important in herbal medicine - you should never exceed the recommended dosages. It is also important to discontinue use of the herbs and consult mainstream medical care if the patient's condition persists or worsens.

Obviously some herbal remedies have value but they also have drawbacks. Even herbs that seem to helpful one person may be dangerous to another - talk to your doctor or pharmacist before using herbs for a serious medical condition, as they may interact with other existing prescription medications or medical conditions that you may have.

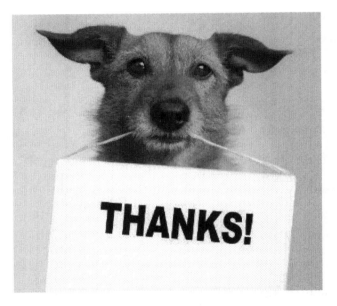

Finally, if you enjoyed this book, then I'd like to ask you for a favour - would you be kind enough to leave a review for this book on Amazon? It would be greatly appreciated!

Click here to leave a review for this book on Amazon!

http://amzn.to/1lgvUAQ

Thank you and good luck!

Check Out My Other Books

Below you'll find some of my other popular books that are popular on Amazon and Kindle as well. Simply click on the links below to check them out.

Mason Jar Meals: Quick and Easy Recipes for Meals on the Go, in a Jar

Canning and Preserving: Everything You Need to Know About How to Can and Preserve Anything!

Eco-Friendly Cleaning: Money Saving Solutions for a Clean, Green, All-Natural, Non-Toxic, Eco-Friendly Home

Herbal Antibiotics & Antivirals: How to Cure Illness with Holistic, All Natural, Herbal Medicines and Remedies

Meditation for Beginners: Learn How to get a Healthy Mind, Body, and Spirit through Meditation

The Sustainable Energy Solution: How to save A LOT of money on your energy bill through renewable energy, sustainable energy, and green living

If the links do not work, for whatever reason, you can simply search for these titles on the Amazon website to find them.

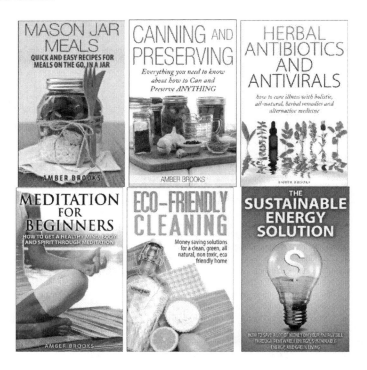

The trademarks that are used are without any consent, and the publication of the trademark is without permission or backing by the trademark owner. All trademarks and brands within this book are for clarifying purposes only and are the owned by the owners themselves, not affiliated with this document.

Made in the USA
Columbia, SC
26 January 2024

30874611R00030